NEW GUINEA SINGING DOG

The Complete Handbook On How To Raising And Caring For New Guinea Singing Dog

CHAD BRUNO

Table of Contents

Introductory

The New Guinea singing dog, abbreviated as "NGSD" or simply "singing dog," is a rare and distinctive domestic dog breed that originated on the island of New Guinea. These dogs are well-known for their unique and beautiful vocalizations, which have been likened to a series of howls, yodels, and whines.

Among the most distinguishing features of the New Guinea singing dog are:

1. The singing dog is well-known for its extensive repertoire of

vocalizations, which it uses to convey meaning. These vocalizations are significantly distinct from the barking of other domesticated dogs and are supposed to mirror the calls of their wild counterparts.

2. These canines, which resemble foxes in size and build, are small to medium in stature. They have a short coat that can be any color or pattern with a wedge-shaped head, upright ears, and a bushy tail.

3. New Guinea singing dogs are notoriously lively and nimble creatures. They are reserved and wary around others, but after being

socialized, they become devoted friends. They are bright and independent, which can make them tough to train.

4. New Guinea singing dogs are elusive in both their native environment and as house pets. In the wild, you'll seek them out in the secluded mountains of New Guinea. The number of purebred NGSDs is low, and they are not widely maintained as pets among captive populations.

Because of the threats posed by habitat degradation, killing, and inbreeding with feral domestic dogs, these dogs are classified as critically endangered in the wild. The purebred New Guinea singing dog is being protected both in zoos and in their native environment through conservation initiatives.

A breed with its own special traits and cultural significance, the New Guinea singing dog is fascinating in its own right and worth learning more about. They are not commonly kept as pets, but have garnered favor among dog lovers and scientists because of their unique traits.

CHAPTER ONE
Personality and Characteristics of Physical Appearance

When compared to other types of domesticated dogs, New Guinea singing dogs (NGSDs) stand out for their unique combination of physical qualities and personality quirks. Here is a rundown of their appearance and personality quirks:

Outer Description:

1. New Guinea singing dogs range in size from little to medium. They typically weigh between 17 to 30 pounds (8 to 14 kg).

2. They have a somewhat pointed nose and a wedge-shaped head. Their pointy ears stand straight up, giving them a fox-like profile.

3. Short and dense, their coat is generally described as "plush." It comes in a wide variety of colors and patterns, such as red, sable, black and tan, and more.

4. **Bushy tail:** NGSDs' tails are typically curled or curved over their backs.

5. **Limbs:** They have well-proportioned limbs, and their feet are tiny and cat-like, which is believed to assist them cross the

rugged terrain in their native habitat.

Character quirks:

1. The distinctive vocalizations of NGSDs are arguably their most well-known feature. They have been given the nickname "singing dog" because to the musicality of their howls, yodels, and whines. These sounds serve a different purpose than barking does in most dog breeds and are utilized for communicating.

2. The New Guinea singing dog is famous for its autonomy. They are confident in who they are and can

rely on themselves to get things done. Although they may be disobedient compared to other dog breeds, their independent nature also makes them creative problem solvers.

3. **Shyness:** NGSDs tend to be naturally wary around humans, especially if they haven't been properly socialized from an early age. They may be reticent or timid around strangers or unfamiliar circumstances.

4. The dogs in this breed are very active and quick on their feet. They are perfectly adapted to surviving in the harsh conditions of their

natural environment. Their athletic qualities make them good climbers and jumpers.

5. Independent, yet Loyal to Their Pack: When raised with humans, NGSDs can be devoted to and protective of their human pack. Strong attachments to their owners are possible.

6. Training a New Guinea singing dog might be difficult because of the breed's stubbornness and individualism. They are not as eager to please as other breeds, therefore they need to be trained with patience and consistency.

7. These canines have a reputation for being naturally inquisitive and eager to discover new things. It's possible that they're naturally curious and like to learn about new places.

It's worth noting that New Guinea singing dogs are quite unusual, and that individuals can exhibit a wide range of personality types. In addition, their wild ancestry and distinct evolutionary history inform their behavior and distinctive features, which classify them as a primitive dog breed. In order to have success with them as pets, they need to be properly socialized and trained.

Permits and Other Legal Matters

New Guinea singing dogs (NGSDs) have different legal considerations and licenses depending on where you live, whether you want to keep one as a pet, and whether you want to participate in a conservation or breeding program. Some broad rules of thumb are as follows:

1. As a Pet to Be Owned:

First and foremost, it's important to find out if owning a non-game species of domesticated animal (NGSD) or exotic pet is prohibited by any state or local laws. Some areas may have limitations or bans on particular breeds or wild animals.

Depending on where you live, and whether or not NGSDs are viewed as a rare or exotic breed, you may be required to obtain a special license or permit in order to acquire one.

• Zoning Regulations zoning regulations in your area may determine whether or not an NGSD can be kept on your property. The number and kind of pets you can keep may be limited by your municipality.

2. Programs for Conservation and Propagation:

More rigorous rules may apply to your work with NGSDs for conservation or breeding purposes, depending on where you live. Among these prerequisites are:

Since NGSDs are a critically endangered species, working with them as part of a conservation program may necessitate the acquisition of wildlife licenses. You might need to engage with governmental or wildlife conservation agencies.

In order to breed NGSDs, you may be required to get a breeding license, and the breeding program may be governed by rules intended to protect the NGSD population.

• CITES: The Convention on International Trade in Endangered Species of Wild Fauna and Flora (CITES) may apply to NGSDs. International commerce in these species is controlled since they are on Appendix II. Importing, exporting, or otherwise conducting business with them necessitates the appropriate licenses and paperwork.

Health and quarantine rules may need to be followed when working with NGSDs in order to limit the transmission of disease and protect the animals.

Before acquiring or working with NGSDs, it is essential to do extensive research and confer with local, regional, and national authorities as well as experts in NGSD conservation and breeding. To protect the animals and follow the law, you must be prepared. As the NGSD population's conservation status changes, rules and permit requirements may also shift, therefore it's important to keep up with the latest developments.

CHAPTER TWO
Preparing a Proper Setting

New Guinea singing dogs (NGSDs) demand special thought while creating an appropriate habitat for them. Since these canines are notoriously free-spirited and energetic, it's crucial to design a home that can keep up with their dynamic lifestyle.

1. Safe and Sound Backyard:

• NGSDs are nimble and can be great climbers and diggers. If you have pets in your yard, make sure they can't go out. It's suggested that a tall fence have a barrier at the bottom to discourage digging.

2. **Free Exploration Zone:**

Give them a lot of room to wander around in. NGSDs are naturally inquisitive and like to learn about the world around them. They may benefit from time spent in a large yard that features a variety of topography and natural components like rocks and trees.

3. **Enrichment:**

• Keep children mentally busy by providing toys, puzzles, and activities that test their problem-solving ability. NGSDs thrive when they have opportunity for mental and physical involvement.

4. Shelter:

• They need some kind of protection from the elements, like a doghouse or a roofed area. NGSDs can survive in a wide range of temperatures, but they still need a safe haven in the event of a heat wave or a cold snap.

5. Socialization:

• NGSDs may experience social anxiety when exposed to novel situations. Introduce children to new experiences and people at an early age to help them develop a tolerance for novelty.

6. **Exercise:**

These dogs are high-energy and require daily walks. Plan for daily walks, playing, and activities to keep them physically active and cognitively engaged.

7. **Confined Spaces:**

If you want to keep your NGSD at home, you need set up secure locations for it to exercise and play. Avoid giving them anything they could choke on or ingest if you can.

8. Instruction and Limits:

• Due to their independent nature, NGSDs require tough yet positive reinforcement-based instruction. Make sure they know what is expected of them by setting firm limits and ground rules.

9. Interaction:

• Make time for your NGSD. Despite their seeming lack of need for human contact, they value friendship.

10. Animal Health:

• It is critical to get them examined by a veterinarian on a regular basis so that any health problems can be caught early and treated. Vaccinations, spaying/neutering (if not used for reproduction), and preventative care should all be considered.

11. Improved Natural Conditions:

Allow children to act on their innate curiosities by giving them space to do so. Their inquisitive minds can be engaged with games of scent, hide-and-seek, and puzzle feeders.

Keep in mind that NGSDs are not a typical breed, so they may require special attention compared to other canine species. Be careful to consult with professionals or NGSD aficionados to get their input as you plan the ideal habitat for these canine eccentrics. It's important to remain dedicated for the long haul, as these dogs can live up to 15 years.

Nutrition and Diet

New Guinea singing dogs (NGSDs) and other domesticated dogs benefit greatly from a well-balanced diet and regular feedings. Like many other dog breeds, NGSDs have special dietary needs that must be met. Here are some suggestions for improving their nutrition:

1. **Premium dog food:**

• Pick a commercial dog food of great quality that is suitable for your dog's age and stage of life (puppy, adult, senior). Look for companies with meat as the primary ingredient and minimum fillers.

2. **Protein:**

• A diet with a moderate to high protein level is recommended for NGSDs. They need protein to keep their muscles and bodies healthy. High-quality protein sources like chicken, steak, or fish are recommended.

3. Fat:

To keep their energy levels up and their skin and coat in good condition, you should make sure they eat a modest amount of healthy fats.

4. Carbohydrates:

• Canines may be carnivores at heart, but they perform well on a diet that includes some starchy foods. But their food shouldn't have too many carbohydrates in it. Choose a dog meal that is high in carbs that the dog can readily digest, such as sweet potatoes or brown rice.

5. **Produce that has just been harvested:**

As a means of supplementing their diet with healthy vitamins and fiber, you can give them fresh fruits and vegetables on a regular basis. Common possibilities include carrots, apples, and green beans.

6. **Throw out the Bad Eats:**

Chocolate, grapes, raisins, onions, garlic, and some fake sweeteners are all poisonous to dogs. These ought to be stored somewhere out of reach.

7. Dietary Restrictions:

• Feed NGSDs according to their age, size, and activity level. If these dogs get too many extra calories, they can become overweight.

8. True Hydration:

Maintain a steady supply of potable water. Their health depends on them staying hydrated.

9. Concerns about Your Diet:

While rare, food allergies and sensitivities do exist among NGSDs. Look out for symptoms like diarrhea or rashes and make dietary changes as needed. If you have concerns about your pet's diet, it's best to make an appointment with a vet.

10. **Supplements:**

• Supplements, such fish oil for omega-3 fatty acids or joint supplements, may be recommended by your veterinarian to improve your pet's overall health.

11. Scheduled, Ongoing Mealtimes:

• Establish a regular eating plan to assist control their digestion and bring structure to their day. Split their daily rations in half or thirds.

12. Talk to Your Vet:

• Your NGSD's health and nutritional needs must be monitored with regular visits to the veterinarian. To find out what food is best for your dog, talk to your vet.

It's important to keep in mind that an NGSD's nutritional demands can fluctuate based on age, activity level, and preexisting diseases. To make sure your NGSD gets the finest nutrition and is healthy throughout its life, it's important to work together with a veterinarian to create a specialized food plan.

CHAPTER THREE
Medical and Animal Services

New Guinea singing dogs (NGSDs) require regular veterinarian treatment and attention to their health as part of proper pet ownership. Like all dog breeds, NGSDs require frequent healthcare to preserve their well-being. Key factors in their well-being and veterinary treatment include:

1. Exams by Veterinarians:

• Take your NGSD in for frequent checkups at the vet. Although annual checkups are the norm, puppies, senior dogs, and dogs with unique health conditions may require more regular visits.

2. **Vaccinations:**

• Get your NGSD up-to-date on all the necessary immunizations, as directed by your vet. Disease prevalence and other factors in a given area may dictate which vaccinations are necessary. Vaccination schedules should be discussed with your veterinarian.

3. **Managing Parasites:**

• Implement a regular deworming and flea/tick prevention regimen for your NGSD. Like other dog breeds, these canines are at risk for parasite infestation.

4. Spaying/Neutering:

• Spaying or neutering may be a good option for your NGSD; talk to your vet about it. This option may depend on their age, health, and your objectives for reproduction.

5. Care for Your Teeth:

• Dental health is vital. The best way to avoid dental problems is to maintain a regular routine of brushing and visiting the dentist.

6. Diet and Weight Control:

• Be sure to keep an eye on your NGSD's weight and feed it a healthy diet. Overeating can cause a variety of health issues, so it's important to exercise caution.

7. Physical Activity and Psychic Challenges:

• Physical and mental well-being depend on regular exercise and cognitive challenge. Do things with them that will stimulate their minds and satisfy their natural inquisitiveness.

8. **Medicine and Health:**

• Keep detailed health records, including vaccination histories, medication records, and any veterinary diagnosis or treatments.

9. **Care in an Emergency:**

• Know where the closest animal hospital that is open 24/7 is located in case of an emergency.

10. Identify any potential health issues that are unique to NGSD breeds. Despite the fact that they are generally healthy canines, it is important to be knowledgeable and proactive. Some potential difficulties could include hip dysplasia, autoimmune illnesses, or hereditary abnormalities.

11. Careful Maintenance:

• NGSDs require regular grooming because of their dense coat. Make sure their nails are trimmed and their ears are clean to avoid infections.

12. Sensitivity to Heat or Cold:

Keep in mind that they can't handle the heat or cold very well. Make sure they have enough protection from the elements.

13. **Socialization:**

• Behavioral disorders and stress-related health issues can be mitigated via early and consistent socialization with other canines and people.

14. **Medicine and Psychology:**

• Keep an eye on how they're feeling emotionally and how they're acting. A veterinarian or dog behaviorist should be consulted if your dog exhibits any anxious, aggressive, or otherwise problematic behaviors.

The key to giving your NGSD a long and healthy life is to take care of its health on a regular basis, both in and out of the vet's office. If you have any queries or concerns regarding the health of your New Guinea singing dog, it is imperative that you contact a veterinarian with expertise in the care of this breed.

Education and Interaction

Raising a well-adjusted and well-behaved New Guinea singing dog (NGSD) relies heavily on training and socializing. These dogs can be independent and wary around new people and situations, so early and continuous training and socialization are crucial for a pleasant and happy bond. Here's how you should go about socializing and training NGSDs:

Training:

1. The best time to start training your NGSD is when he or she is still a young puppy. Their behavior can be molded more easily through early teaching.

2. Treats, praise, and rewards are all examples of positive reinforcement that can be used to inspire and reinforce the behaviors you want to see more of. NGSDs are bright, and they learn quickly and easily from praise and encouragement.

3. Maintain a steady approach to training. Set clear boundaries and regulations, and ensure that all family members and caregivers follow the same norms.

4. Sit, stay, come, and leash training are all fundamental instructions that must be taught. These cues will help keep your dog safe and give him a sense of direction in a variety of settings.

5. Leash training is essential because NGSDs are naturally curious. A well-mannered NGSD on a leash is far less of a liability.

6. The importance of early socialization cannot be overstated. You may help your NGSD overcome shyness and dread of new experiences by exposing it to a wide range of people, canines, and settings. Participating in puppy socialization sessions may prove useful.

7. To encourage excellent behavior and handle any unique training requirements, you may choose to enroll your NGSD in obedience lessons or work with a professional dog trainer.

Socialization:

1. Get your NGSD out and about as soon as possible. Socialization is most effective between the ages of 3 and 14 weeks, but it is important at any age.

2. Introduce your dog to individuals of varied ages, genders, and physical traits. Promote pleasant encounters by rewarding good behavior with snacks and compliments.

3. Let your NGSD play with other well-mannered dogs who have all had their vaccinations. This teaches

them how to interact with other dogs properly.

4. Expose your dog to a wide range of situations, from urban and rural locations to parks. This will help children adjust to varied conditions.

5. Encourage children to use all of their senses, including touch, sight, sound, and scent. Anxiety and terror can be alleviated with positive exposure to a wide range of stimuli.

6. Reward your NGSD with goodies and praise when they behave calmly and confidently in novel settings. Facilitate happy and

successful interactions in their social lives.

7. Increase the level of challenge encountered throughout socialization events over time. It's best to ease into more difficult situations rather than jumping right in.

8. Keep an eye out for the NGSD's physical manifestations of stress. If they begin to show indications of anxiety, it's best to remove them from the scenario and try again at a later time or in a less stressful environment.

Keep in mind that every NGSD is an individual with potentially different requirements for socializing and training. Take your time, stay consistent, and be flexible. Your NGSD will flourish as a well-adjusted and self-assured pet if you start socializing and teaching him or her as a puppy. In the event that you run into any difficulties, it may be helpful to seek the advice of a professional dog trainer who has expertise working with NGSDs.

Reproduction and Breeding

Due to their highly endangered status in the wild, New Guinea singing dogs (NGSDs) require a cautious and responsible approach to breeding and reproduction. If you want to breed NGSDs, you need know all about their unique requirements, health concerns, and the significance of protecting the breed's genetic variety.

1. Both the male and female NGSDs need to pass a health screening before they can mate. This involves regular veterinarian check-ups, immunizations, and screens for genetic and hereditary disorders that may impact the breed.

2. Given the small size of the NGSD gene pool, it is crucial to preserve and protect the breed's genetic

variety. You should think about the genetic variety and history of the dogs you wish to breed to prevent health issues caused by inbreeding.

3. Health Clearances: Both male and female NGSDs need to have completed the necessary health clearances, which may include tests for hereditary disorders, vision screenings, and evaluations of the hips and elbows. These checks are important for making sure the babies are healthy.

4. When selecting breeding candidates, look for animals that exhibit desirable behavioral traits and correspond to the breed

standard. Think about their family tree and how they can help the NGSD breed survive.

5. Timing is essential for productive breeding. Female NGSDs enter heat (estrus) twice a year, on average. The best period for mating can be determined with the advice of a vet or a knowledgeable breeder.

6. Breeding NGSDs requires supervision during the mating procedure because the animals' independence can make them less cooperative. Managing or consulting an expert may be necessary.

7. Whelping and Pregnancy Care Give the pregnant female enough of food and regular veterinary checkups. Make sure the area where the puppies will be born is clean and secure in preparation for the whelping process.

8. Care for Puppies: Puppies with NGSD require extra attention. Introduce them to new people and activities at an early age, keep an eye on their health, and feed them well. Think about how to best ensure the safety of the mother and her offspring.

9. Place the puppies with caring people who know what they're

doing. Carefully vet prospective owners to make sure they can provide a safe, happy home for the NGSDs.

10. Know your local laws and obtain the necessary licenses before bringing any NGSDs home to breed. It's possible that unusual and rare dog breeds are subject to additional rules in certain areas.

11. Since NGSDs are now considered extinct, breeding them should only be done for ethical reasons (such as the continuation and betterment of the breed) and not for financial gain. Ethical

breeding is vital for the long-term wellbeing of the breed.

Responsible NGSD breeding is essential for the survival of the breed and the development of healthy, well-adjusted dogs. Expert advice from breeders, geneticists, and veterinarians familiar with NGSDs is worth seeking out at every stage of the breeding process.

Conclusion

New Guinea singing dogs (NGSDs) are an exotic and unusual breed with specific needs in terms of lifestyle and upkeep. Understanding and meeting the demands of NGSDs is an important part of responsible ownership. What you need to know is as follows:

1. **Distinguishing Features:** NGSDs are well-known for their beautiful singing voices, dexterity, freedom, and wariness in unfamiliar settings and with unfamiliar people. They have a fox-like look with a thick coat and a bushy tail.

2. A balanced diet, regular veterinary examinations, immunizations, and parasite control are all crucial to their health. Seek the advice of a vet familiar with NGSDs if you're

worried about any potential health issues.

3. Socialization and training are equally important for NGSDs, and should begin at an early age. They can be shaped into well-behaved, self-assured companions with the use of positive reinforcement techniques, socialization, and cerebral stimulation.

4. Indoors or out, the setting should be safe, interesting, and accommodating to NGSDs. Fencing in the yard, providing stimulating activities, and keeping the animal out of the cold are all essential.

5. Breeding and Reproduction: Breeding NGSDs should be undertaken with caution, concentrating on health, genetic variety, and preservation of the breed. The survival of this species depends on the use of ethical breeding techniques.

6. Keep in mind that the laws and licenses necessary to possess and breed NGSDs may differ depending on where you live.

7. Conservation: NGSDs are highly endangered in the wild. The survival of the species depends on our ability to conserve and safeguard it.

The care and survival of the NGSD breed depends on the owner's expertise, experience, and devotion. Care for these extraordinary dogs is best approached with the help of specialists and seasoned NGSD aficionados.

THE END

www.ingramcontent.com/pod-product-compliance
Lightning Source LLC
Chambersburg PA
CBHW070821290526
45795CB00002B/797